I0696523

# Living With Heart Disease

## A Guide to Lifelong Cardiovascular Health

Rossana Lewis

All rights reserved. No part of this publication may be reproduced, distributed or transmitted in any form or by any means, including photocopying, recording or other electronic or mechanical methods without the prior written permission of the publisher, except in the case of brief quotations embodied in critical reviews and certain other non-commercial uses permitted by copyright law.

For permission requests, write to the publisher at the address below.

Email: rossanalewis01@gmail.com

# TABLE OF CONTENT


Chapter 1: The Heart and Cardiovascular System

1.1 Anatomy and Function

1.2 Common Heart Conditions

Chapter 2: Risk Factors and Prevention

2.1 Identifying Risk Factors

2.2 Strategies for Prevention

Chapter 3: Diagnosis and Diagnostic Tests

Chapter 4: Treatment Approaches

4.1 Medications

4.2 Surgical and Interventional Options

Chapter 5: Heart-Healthy Diet

5.1 Nutritional Strategies

5.2 Meal Planning and Recipes

Chapter 6: Exercise and Physical Activity

6.1 The Benefits of Regular Exercise

6.2 Developing a Fitness Plan

Chapter 7: Stress Management and Mental Wellness

7.1 Stress's Impact on the Heart

7.2 Coping Strategies and Mind-Body Practices

Chapter 8: Medication Management

8.1 Understanding Your Medications

8.2 Adherence and Side Effects

Chapter 9: Cardiac Rehabilitation

9.1 The Role of Cardiac Rehab

9.2 Participating in Your Recovery

Chapter 10: Survivorship and Lifestyle Beyond Heart Disease

10.1 Embracing a Heart-Healthy Lifestyle

10.2 Monitoring and Preventing Recurrence

# Chapter 1: The Heart and Cardiovascular System

## 1.1 Anatomy and Function

The heart is a fist-sized organ that pumps blood throughout your body. It's the primary organ of your circulatory system.

It contains four main sections (chambers) made of muscle and powered by electrical impulses. Your brain and nervous system direct your heart's function.

The heart is located in the front of the chest. It sits slightly behind and to the left of your sternum (breastbone). The ribcage protects your heart.

What is the function of the Heart?

The heart's main function is to move blood throughout the body. It also controls the rhythm and speed of the heart rate.

The heart also maintains your blood pressure.

It has parts which makes up its anatomy, which are:

The Heart Walls: which are the muscles that contract (squeeze) and relax to send blood throughout the body. A layer of muscular tissue called the septum divides the heart walls into the left and right sides. The heart wall has three layers: the endocardium also known as the inner layer, the myocardium also known as the muscular middle layer and the epicardium also known as the protective outer layer. The epicardium is one layer of the pericardium. The pericardium is a protective sac that covers the entire heart. It produces fluid to lubricate the heart and keep it from rubbing against other organs.

The Heart Chambers: is divided into four chambers. You have two chambers on the top (atrium, plural atria) and two on the bottom (ventricles), one on each side of the heart.

The Heart Valves: are like doors between the heart chambers. They open and close to allow blood to flow through. The atrioventricular (AV) valves open between your upper and lower heart chambers. They include: tricuspid valve and mitral valve while the semilunar (SL) valves open when blood flows out of the ventricles and they include: aortic valve and pulmonary valve.

Blood Vessels: the heart pumps blood through three types of blood vessels: arteries, veins and capillaries.

Electrical Conduction System: the heart's conduction system is like the electrical wiring of a house. It controls the rhythm and pace of your heartbeat. It includes: sinoatrial (SA) node and atrioventricular (AV) node.

## 1.2 Common Heart Conditions

There are many different heart conditions and problems which are collectively called heart disease.

It's always best to discuss your heart condition with your health professional or heart specialist who can advise you on the correct diagnosis and name of your condition and treatment plan.

Heart disease and different conditions affect the heart's ability to work efficiently. It can be worrying and confusing to be diagnosed with a heart condition, but there's a lot of information and support available to you. Sometimes understanding what is happening can help you worry less.

Coronary Artery Disease (CAD): CAD is the most common heart problem. With CAD, you may get blockages in your coronary arteries, the vessels that supply blood to your heart. That can lead to a decrease in the flow of blood to your heart muscle, keeping it from getting the oxygen it needs. The disease usually starts as a result of atherosclerosis, a condition sometimes called hardening of the arteries. Coronary heart disease can give you pain in your chest, called angina, or lead to a heart attack.

Heart Arrhythmias: When you have an arrhythmia, your heart has an irregular beating pattern. Serious arrhythmias often develop from other heart problems but may also happen on their own.

Heart Valve Disease: Your heart has four valves that open and close to direct blood flow between your heart's four chambers, the lungs, and blood vessels. An abnormality could make it hard for a valve to open and close the right way. When that happens, your blood flow could be blocked or blood can leak. Your valve may not open and close right. The causes of heart valve problems include infections such as rheumatic fever, congenital heart disease, high blood pressure, coronary artery disease, or as a result of a heart attack.

Pericardial Disease: Any disease of the pericardium, the sac that surrounds your heart, is called a pericardial disease. One of the more common diseases is pericarditis or inflammation of the pericardium. It's usually caused by an infection with a virus, inflammatory diseases such as lupus or rheumatoid arthritis, or injury to your pericardium. Pericarditis often follows open heart surgery.

Cardiomyopathy (Heart Muscle Disease): Cardiomyopathy is a disease of your heart muscle, or myocardium. It gets stretched, thickened, or stiff. Your heart may get too weak to pump well.

There are many possible causes of the disease, including genetic heart conditions, reactions to certain drugs or toxins (such as alcohol), and infections from a virus. Sometimes, chemotherapy causes cardiomyopathy. Many times, doctors can't find the exact cause.

Congenital Heart Disease: Congenital heart disease happens when something goes wrong while the heart is forming in a baby that's still in the womb. Heart abnormality sometimes leads to problems right after birth, but other times there aren't any symptoms until you become an adult. Septal abnormalities are among the most common congenital heart problems. These are holes in the wall that separates the left and right sides of your heart. You can get a procedure to patch the hole. Another type of abnormality is called pulmonary stenosis. A narrow valve causes a decrease in the flow of blood to your lungs. A procedure or surgery can open or replace the valve.

In some babies, a small blood vessel known as the ductus arteriosus doesn't close up at birth as it should. When this happens, some blood leaks back into the pulmonary artery, which puts strain on your heart. Doctors can treat this with surgery or a procedure or sometimes with medication.

# Chapter 2: Risk Factors and Prevention

## 2.1 Identifying Risk Factors

There are risk factors for heart disease that you have control over and others that you don't. Uncontrollable risk factors for heart disease include:

- Being male
- Older age
- Family history of heart disease
- Being postmenopausal
- Race (African American, Native American, and Mexican American people are more likely to have heart disease)

Heart disease risk factors that you can control revolve around lifestyle. These include:

- Smoking

- Unhealthy cholesterol numbers

- Uncontrolled high blood pressure

- Physical inactivity

- Obesity (having a BMI greater than 25)

- Uncontrolled diabetes

- Uncontrolled stress, depression, and anger

- Poor diet

- Alcohol use

## 2.2 Strategies for Prevention

Research shows heart disease may be preventable more than half the time with simple changes in lifestyle. Besides lowering your risk for heart attack and stroke, these changes often can improve your overall physical and mental health. Here are some ways you can change lifestyle factors to reduce your risk of heart disease:

Quit Smoking: Smoking is the most preventable risk factor. Smokers have more than twice the risk of heart attack as nonsmokers and are much more likely to die from them. If you smoke, quit. Better yet, don't start smoking in the first place. Even if you don't smoke, constant exposure to other people's cigarette smoke (secondhand smoke) raises your risk of heart disease.

Improve Cholesterol Levels: Your risk for heart disease increases with unhealthy cholesterol numbers. The right levels can vary somewhat depending on your age, sex, overall health, and family health history. Ask your doctor about the right levels for you. In general, though, your levels should be as follows:

- Total cholesterol: less than 200 mg/dL

- "Good," or HDL, cholesterol: 60 mg/dL or greater

- "Bad," or LDL, cholesterol: less than 100 mg/dL

- Triglycerides: less than 150 mg/dL

A diet low in cholesterol, saturated and trans fats, and simple sugars, and high in complex carbohydrates can help lower cholesterol levels in some people. Regular exercise will also help lower "bad" cholesterol and raise "good" cholesterol in some cases.

If that's not enough, your doctor may suggest a cholesterol medication, like a statin, to help lower levels.

Control High Blood Pressure: About 67 million people in the U.S. have high blood pressure, making it the most common risk factor for heart disease. Nearly 1 in 3 adults have systolic blood pressure (the upper number) over 130, and/or diastolic blood pressure (the lower number) over 80, which is the definition of high blood pressure. Your doctor will assess your blood pressure numbers in light of your overall health, lifestyle, and other risk factors. You and your doctor can come up with a plan to help control blood pressure through diet, exercise, weight management, and if needed, medication.

Control Diabetes: if not properly controlled, diabetes can lead to heart disease and heart damage, including heart attacks. Control diabetes through a healthy diet, exercise, maintaining a healthy weight, and medication as prescribed by your doctor.

Get Active: People who don't exercise have higher rates of heart disease compared to people who perform even moderate amounts of physical activity. A bit of light gardening or walking can lower your risk of heart disease.

Most people should exercise 30 minutes a day, at moderate intensity, on most days. More vigorous exercise could help even more, but talk to your doctor first. Try to use large muscle groups and get your heart rate up. Aerobic activities that raise your heart rate include brisk walking, cycling, swimming, jumping rope, and jogging. You can also lift weights to increase strength and muscle endurance. If motivation is a problem, make an exercise menu. Pick a couple of activities that sound like fun. That way, you always have some choices. Consult your doctor before starting any exercise program, especially if you have underlying health conditions or haven't exercised in a while.

Eat Right: Eat a heart-healthy diet low in sodium, saturated fat, trans fat, cholesterol, and refined sugars. Try to increase your intake of foods rich in vitamins and other nutrients, especially antioxidants, which may lower your risk for heart disease. Also eat plant-based foods such as fruits and vegetables, nuts, and whole grains.

Rethink Your Drink: Limit alcohol. Moderate drinking may be OK, but more than that isn't good for your heart health. What's moderate drinking? Up to one glass a day for women, and up to two glasses a day for men.

Maintain a Healthy Weight: Obesity by itself could raise your risk for heart disease. In addition, excess weight puts strain on your heart and often raises your risk of other heart disease risk factors like diabetes, high blood pressure, and high cholesterol. A balanced diet and regular exercise can help you keep a healthy weight. Talk to your doctor if you need a safe plan for weight loss or if you want to figure out the right body weight for your heart health.

Manage Stress: Poorly controlled stress and anger can worsen heart disease.

Talk to Your Doctor: Discuss your lifestyle as well as your family's medical history with your doctor. Together you'll be able to come up with a plan best suited to your needs.

# Chapter 3: Diagnosis and Diagnostic Test

Cardiovascular diseases are diagnosed using an array of laboratory tests and imaging studies. The primary part of diagnosis is medical and family histories of the patient, risk factors, physical examination and coordination of these findings with the results from tests and procedures.

Some of the common tests used to diagnose cardiovascular diseases include:

Blood Tests: Laboratory tests are used to detect the risk factors for heart diseases. These include detection of the fats, cholesterol and lipid components of blood including LDL, HDL, Triglycerides.

Blood sugar and Glycosylated hemoglobin is measured for detection of diabetes. C-reactive protein (CRP) and other protein markers like Apolipoprotein A1 and B are used to detect inflammation that may lead to heart diseases.

During a heart attack, heart muscle cells die and release proteins into the bloodstream. Blood tests can measure the amount of these proteins in the bloodstream. High levels of these proteins are a sign of a recent heart attack.

One of the markers of heart attack is the Cardiac Troponin-T. Other biomarkers include fibrinogen and PAI-1, high levels of homocysteine, elevated asymmetric dimethylarginine and elevated brain natriuretic peptide (also known as B-type) (BNP).

Electrocardiogram(EKG/ECG): This is a simple and a painless test that records the heart's electrical activity. The patient is strapped to the instrument with several patches or leads placed over his or her chest, wrists and ankles. A small portable machine records the activities of the heart on a strip of graph paper.

The test shows how fast the heart is beating and its rhythm. The strength and timing of the electrical signals as they pass through the heart are also seen. An EKG/ECG can help detect a heart attack, attacks of angina, arrhythmias etc.

Stress Testing: For this test, the patient is made to work hard e.g. run on a treadmill or exercise while the leads of ECG/EKG are placed over their body. Those who cannot exercise are given pills to raise their heart rate. The test detects the effects of the exercise on the heart. In patients with atherosclerosis and coronary heart diseases the arteries that are narrowed by plaques cannot supply adequate blood to the heart muscles while it is beating faster. This may lead to shortness of breath and chest pain. The EKG/ECG pattern, arrhythmias etc. also show the possibility of a coronary artery disease.

Echocardiography: This test uses sound waves to create a moving picture of the heart. This is also a painless test where a probe is rolled over the chest and the machine creates the image of the heart on the monitor. This provides information on the shape, size, workings, valves and chambers of the heart. Echocardiography may also be combined with Doppler to show the areas of poor blood supply to the heart. It shows the areas of the heart muscle that are not contracting normally, and previous injury to the heart muscle.

Coronary Angiography and Cardiac Catheterization: This test is an invasive test. A dye is injected into the veins to reach the coronary arteries. This is done via coronary catheterization. Thereafter detailed pictures of the blood vessels of the heart are taken using special imaging methods. This is called coronary angiography.

Cardiac catheterization involves threading of a thin, flexible tube called a catheter via blood vessels in the arm, groin (upper thigh), or neck. The tube is inserted under imagin guidance till it reaches the heart. Coronary angiography detects blockages in the large coronary arteries.

Chest X Ray: This is a test that shows the shape and size of the heart lungs and major blood vessels. This is a test seldom used in diagnosis of heart diseases as it does not provide added information over echocardiography and other imaging studies.

Electron-Beam Computed Tomography or EBCT: helps to detect the calcium deposits or calcifications in the walls of the coronary arteries. These are early markers of atherosclerosis and coronary heart disease. This is not a routine test in coronary heart disease.

Cardiac MRI: Cardiac MRI (magnetic resonance imaging) that uses radio waves, magnets, and a computer to create pictures of the heart. This gives a 3D image of the moving as well as still pictures of the heart.

# Chapter 4: Treatment Approaches

## 4.1 Medications

If you recently had a heart attack or been diagnosed with a heart disease, it's likely you were prescribed medication. It's important to understand what heart-related medications do, how to take them safely and recognize possible side effects.

Remember your doctor and pharmacist are your best sources of information when it comes to your medications.

Heart medications are given to treat heart conditions, manage symptoms and reduce the risk of future heart and vascular events, such as heart attack, heart failure, and stroke. If you are a heart patient, the type of medication you receive will depend on your diagnosis, other conditions you may have, as well as your age and lifestyle.

The following are some of the most common heart medications:

Aspirin: Blood clots can block the flow of blood through the arteries and lead to heart attack or stroke. Aspirin is the most common antiplatelet agent given to prevent blood clots. It can reduce inflammation associated with heart disease.

Physicians prescribe a daily aspirin to patients who have had a prior heart attack, had a stent implanted in the coronary arteries or legs and patients who've had a prior stroke or valve replacement.

After a heart attack and stenting procedure, patients are recommended to take and prescribed an additional antiplatelet medication to help prevent clots. This second clot-preventing medication is taken for a certain period of time that your physician determines is best for you. In most cases, it is not lifelong. Examples include clopidogrel (Plavix), ticagrelor (Brilinta), and prasugrel (Effient).

ACE Inhibitors or ARBs: Angiotensin converting enzyme (ACE) inhibitors and angiotensin receptor blockers (ARBs) dilate, or widen, blood vessels. This helps improve the flow of blood, eases the demands on the heart and lowers blood pressure.

These drugs are often given for high blood pressure and heart failure. They help decrease the risk of heart attack or stroke in people with heart disease. When given after a heart attack, they help prevent heart damage and future heart attacks.

Antiarrhythmics: People with abnormal heart rhythms may be prescribed antiarrhythmic medications. They may have hearts that beat too quickly, too slowly, or irregularly. These drugs help regulate the heart's electrical activity so that the heart beats normally.

They may be used alone or combined with procedures, such as an ablation, or devices, such as pacemakers and/or internal cardiac defibrillators to treat the most concerning rhythm problems of the heart.

Anticoagulants (blood thinners): Anticoagulants are often called blood thinners but they don't actually thin your blood. They help prevent blood from coagulating or clotting.

They're often taken by people who've had heart attacks, have artificial mechanical heart valves, or atrial fibrillation. The most common form of these drugs includes warfarin (Coumadin), rivaroxaban (Xarelto), dabigatran (Pradaxa) and apixaban (Eliquis).

Beta Blockers: Beta blockers are often prescribed after a heart attack to help the heart recover. They minimize the effects of harmful substances produced as a result of heart failure. Some can also help improve the heart's ability to pump blood. Others may be given to treat high blood pressure, angina and abnormal heart rhythms.

Common beta blockers include carvedilol (Coreg), nebivolol (Bystolic), and metoprolol (Toprol).

Calcium channel blockers: Calcium channel blockers decrease the heart's workload by increasing its supply of blood and oxygen. They do this by preventing calcium from entering the cells of the heart and arteries. They can help treat high blood pressure, abnormal heart rhythms and angina.

They are often given to people who cannot take beta blockers and include verapamil (Verelan) and diltiazem (Cardizem).

Statins: Statins help to lower the levels of low-density lipoprotein (LDL) cholesterol ("bad" cholesterol) in the blood. They can also lower triglyceride levels, which are another type of normal fat in the blood that when elevated increases the risk of atherosclerosis (plaque build up).

Statins decrease bad cholesterol production in the liver and inflammation in cholesterol plaques. Common statins include atorvastatin (Lipitor) and rosuvastatin (Crestor).

## 4.2 Surgery and Interventional Options

Heart-related problems do not always require surgery. Sometimes they can be addressed with lifestyle changes, medications, or nonsurgical procedures. For example, catheter ablation uses energy to make small scars in your heart tissue to prevent abnormal electrical signals from moving through your heart. Coronary angioplasty is a minimally invasive procedure in which a stent is inserted into a narrowed or blocked coronary artery to hold it open. Nonetheless, surgery is often needed to address problems such as heart failure, plaque buildup that partially or totally blocks blood flow in a coronary artery, faulty heart valves, dilated or diseased major blood vessels (such as the aorta), and abnormal heart rhythms.

The types of surgery includes:

Coronary Artery Bypass Grafting (CABG): In CABG the most common type of heart surgery, the surgeon takes a healthy artery or vein from elsewhere in your body and connects it to supply blood past the blocked coronary artery. The grafted artery or vein bypasses the blocked portion of the coronary artery, creating a new path for blood to flow to the heart muscle. Often, this is done for more than one coronary artery during the same surgery. CABG is sometimes referred to as heart bypass or coronary artery bypass surgery.

Heart Valve Repair or Replacement: Surgeons either repair the valve or replace it with an artificial valve or with a biological valve made from pig, cow, or human heart tissue. One repair option is to insert a catheter through a large blood vessel, guide it to the heart, and inflate and deflate a small balloon at the tip of the catheter to widen a narrow valve.

Insertion of a Pacemaker or an Implantable Cardioverter Defibrillator (ICD): Medicine is usually the first treatment option for arrhythmia, a condition in which the heart beats too fast, too slow or with an irregular rhythm. If medication does not work, a surgeon may implant a pacemaker under the skin of the chest or abdomen, with wires that connect it to the heart chambers. The device uses electrical pulses to control the heart rhythm when a sensor detects that it is abnormal. An ICD works similarly, but it sends an electric shock to restore a normal rhythm when it detects a dangerous arrhythmia.

Maze Surgery: The surgeon creates a pattern of scar tissue within the upper chambers of the heart to redirect electrical signals along a controlled path to the lower heart chambers. The surgery blocks the stray electrical signals that cause atrial fibrillation, the most common type of serious arrhythmia.

Aneurysm Repair: A weak section of the artery or heart wall is replaced with a patch or graft to repair a balloon-like bulge in the artery or wall of the heart muscle.

Heart Transplant: The diseased heart is removed and replaced with a healthy heart from a deceased donor.

Insertion of a Ventricular Assist Device (VAD) or Total Artificial Heart (TAH): A VAD is a mechanical pump that supports heart function and blood flow. A TAH replaces the two lower chambers of the heart.

# Chapter 5: Heart-Healthy Diets

## 5.1 Nutritional Strategies

Following these nutritional strategies can help you reduce or even eliminate some risk factors.

Choose Fat Calories Wisely: Research has revealed that the total amount of fat you eat really isn't linked to heart disease; it's the type of fat you consume that has the greatest influence. Two unhealthy fats, including saturated and trans fats, raise blood cholesterol and increase the risk for cardiovascular disease. However, two very different types of fat — monounsaturated and polyunsaturated fats — do just the opposite.

Limit Dietary Cholesterol: Because cholesterol is made from the liver, it is only found in foods of animal origin (not in plant-based foods). For most people, the amount of cholesterol in the diet has a modest impact on their blood cholesterol levels. However, there are many people whose blood cholesterol levels fluctuate very strongly with the amount of cholesterol eaten. In addition, cholesterol in the diet greatly affects people who have diabetes.

It is important for everyone to make an effort to limit total dietary cholesterol. If you have high cholesterol, limit your daily dietary cholesterol to 200 milligrams; if you have normal cholesterol levels, limit to 300 milligrams daily.

Get Your Daily Fiber Boost: As part of a healthy diet, fiber can reduce cholesterol. Dietary fiber is a type of carbohydrate that the body cannot digest. It's found primarily in whole grains, fruits, vegetables and beans. As fiber passes through the body, it affects the way the body digests foods and absorbs nutrients.

A diet rich in fiber has health benefits beyond cholesterol control: it helps control blood sugar, promote regularity, prevent gastrointestinal disease and helps in weight management.

Increase Fruits, Vegetables, Legumes and Nuts: Only three percent of Americans consume the recommended amount of fruits, vegetables, legumes and grains recommended by health professionals. To maximize your intake of heart-disease-fighting antioxidants, vitamins, minerals, protein and dietary fiber, adopt the following three strategies.

Substitute Plant Protein for Animal Protein: Increase plant sources of protein and start reducing your intake of animal protein. Research shows this can have a positive overall impact on heart health. Substituting non-meat sources of protein for meat significantly reduces saturated fat and cholesterol and boosts heart-disease-fighting fiber, vitamins, minerals and antioxidants.

Distribute Meals and Snacks: Skipping meals is not recommended. Small, frequent meals and snacks appear to promote weight loss and maintenance and give you an opportunity to consume important nutrients throughout the day. Skipping meals only lowers metabolism and deprives you of key nutrients. Researchers have found that people who balance their calories into four to six small meals each day have lower cholesterol levels.

## 5.2 Meal Planning and Recipes

Following a heart-healthy diet if you're diagnosed with a heart disease is just the right step to recovery. This meal plan is for you! Recipes are lower in sodium and saturated fat, higher in fiber and packed with fresh fruits and veggies.

|  | Breakfast | Lunch | Dinner |
|---|---|---|---|
| Day 1 | Spiced Blueberry Quinoa | Waldorf Turkey Pitas | Chicken with Citrus Chimichurri Sauce |

|        | Breakfast | Lunch | Dinner |
| --- | --- | --- | --- |
| Day 2 | Whole Wheat Pancakes | Contest-Winning Easy Minestrone | Salmon with Horseradish Pistachio Crust |
| Day 3 | Sausage-Egg Burritos | Lemony Garbanzo Salad | Pepper Steak with Potatoes |
| Day 4 | Get-Up-and-Go Granola | Hummus & Veggie Wrap-Up | Turkey Medallions with Tomato Salad |

|  | Breakfast | Lunch | Dinner |
| --- | --- | --- | --- |
| Day 5 | Breakfast Sweet Potatoes | Turkey Salsa Bowls with Tortilla Wedges | Vegetarian Black Bean Pasta |
| Day 6 | Overnight Oatmeal | Chicken and Spinach Pasta Salad | Cod and Asparagus Bake |

# Chapter 6: Exercise and Physical Activity

## 6.1 The Benefits of Regular Exercise

Understanding just how physical activity benefits your heart can be a strong motivation to get moving more.

Exercise Lowers Blood Pressure: Exercise works like beta-blocker medication to slow the heart rate and lower blood pressure (at rest and also when exercising). High blood pressure is a major risk factor for heart disease.

Weight Control: Especially when combined with a smart diet, being physically active is an essential component for losing weight and even more important for keeping it off which in turn helps optimize heart health. Being overweight puts stress on the heart and is a risk factor for heart disease and stroke.

Strengthen Muscles: A combination of aerobic workouts (which, depending on your fitness level, can include walking, running, swimming, and other vigorous heart-pumping exercise) and strength training (weight lifting, resistance training) is considered best for heart health. These exercises improve the muscles' ability to draw oxygen from the circulating blood. That reduces the need for the heart, a muscular organ itself, to work harder to pump more blood to the muscles, whatever your age.

Help Quit Smoking: As smokers become more fit, they often quit. And people who are fit in the first place are less likely to ever start smoking, which is one of the top risk factors for heart disease because it damages the structure and function of blood vessels.

Slow the Development of Diabetes: when combined with strength training, regular aerobic exercise such as cycling, brisk walking, or swimming can reduce the risk of developing diabetes by over 50% by allowing the muscles to better process glycogen, a fuel for energy, which when impaired, leads to excessive blood sugars, and thus diabetes.

Lowers Stress: Stress hormones can put an extra burden on the heart. Exercise, whether aerobic (like running), resistance-oriented (like weight training) or flexibility-focused (like yoga) can help you relax and ease stress.

Reduces Inflammation: With regular exercise, chronic inflammation is reduced as the body adapts to the challenge of exercise on many bodily systems. This is an important factor for reducing the adverse effects of many of the diseases just mentioned.

## 6.2 Developing a Fitness Plan

Exercise is one of the most important things you can do for your heart health. Physical activity helps you live longer and reduces the risk of dying from heart disease by 50%. But after you've been diagnosed with heart disease, you may feel scared and uncertain. Where do you start? How much activity is healthy and safe? For many people, it is easy to start with walking. Below is an example of a walking program. Walk in the hallway, walk the length of your driveway, walk in the mall, walk a block, walk for 10 minutes.

Remember you are starting slow and easy. You may need to plan rest areas or places to stop and sit along the way.

|  | Number of Days | Warm Up | Training Period | Cool Down |
| --- | --- | --- | --- | --- |
| Week1 | Every second day | Nil | 10 minutes walk at an easy pace | Nil |

|  | Number of Days | Warm Up | Training Period | Cool Down |
| --- | --- | --- | --- | --- |
| Week 2 | Every second day | 5min easy walk | 10 minutes walk at a faster rate | 5 minutes easy walk |
| Week 3 | 4 times a week | 5 minutes east walk | 15 minutes walk at a faster pace | 5 minutes easy walk and stretches |

| | Number of Days | Warm Up | Training Period | Cool Down |
|---|---|---|---|---|
| Week 4 | 4 times a week | 5 minutes easy walk | 20 minutes walk at a faster pace | 5 minutes easy walk and stretches |
| Week 5&6 | At Least 5 days a week | 10 minutes easy walk | 25-30 minutes walk at a faster | 5 minutes easy walk and stretche |

|  | Number of Days | Warm Up | Training Period | Cool Down |
| --- | --- | --- | --- | --- |
|  |  |  | pace. Start to pump or swing arms. Walk up gentle hills, moving slightly forward | s for each walk |

# Chapter 7: Stress Management and Mental Wellness

## 7.1 Stress' Impact on the Heart

Stress has become a regular and permanent companion for many people in today's fast-paced world. It's crucial to realize that not all stress is negative; in fact, some types of stress can be inspiring and even helpful. The "fight or flight" response, a physiological response that causes the production of stress hormones like cortisol and adrenaline, is triggered when you are faced with a stressful scenario. This reaction gets your body ready to deal with the perceived threat by raising your heart rate, narrowing your blood vessels, and concentrating on getting oxygen and nutrients to your muscles and brain so you can take rapid action.

Stress can be short-term or chronic.

Short-term stress, such as that felt during urgent events, is typically regarded as normal and helpful. Performance, awareness, and problem-solving skills can all be improved. Chronic stress, which is frequently linked to on-going life issues, can, however, be harmful to health. It puts the heart and blood vessels under strain by causing a prolonged rise in blood pressure, a major risk factor for heart disease. Additionally, it can cause inflammation to spread throughout the body, particularly the arteries, which aids in the onset and development of atherosclerosis.

The impact of stress on the heart is multifaceted. Chronic stress can lead to high blood pressure, which increases the risk of heart attacks and strokes. It can also promote inflammation, a key contributor to atherosclerosis. Stress can disrupt the heart's rhythm, leading to arrhythmias like atrial fibrillation, which can further increase the risk of stroke and other heart-related complications. Additionally, stress hormones can encourage the formation of blood clots, which can obstruct blood flow in the arteries and lead to heart attacks. Lastly, individuals under chronic stress may resort to unhealthy coping behaviors like overeating, smoking, or excessive alcohol consumption, all of which can contribute to the development of heart disease.

## 7.2 Coping Strategies and Mind-Body Practices

It's key to recognize stressful situations as they occur because it allows you to focus on managing how you react. We all need to know when to close our eyes and take a deep breath when we feel tension rising.

The following are mind-body practices and coping strategies you need for stress management:

Rebalance Work and Home: All work and no play? If you're spending too much time at the office, intentionally put more dates in your calendar to enjoy time for fun, either alone or with others.

Get Regular Exercise:Moving your body on a regular basis balances the nervous system and increases blood circulation, helping to flush out stress hormones. Even a daily 20-minute walk makes a difference. Any kind of exercise can lower stress and improve your mood, just pick activities that you enjoy and make it a regular habit.

Eat Well and Limit Alcohol and Stimulants: Alcohol, nicotine and caffeine may temporarily relieve stress but have negative health impacts and can make stress worse in the long run. Well-nourished bodies cope better, so start with a good breakfast, add more organic fruits and vegetables for a well-balanced diet, avoid processed foods and sugar, try herbal tea and drink more water.

Connect with Supportive People: Talking face to face with another person releases hormones that reduce stress. Lean on those good listeners in your life.

Carve Out Hobby Time: Do you enjoy gardening, reading, listening to music or some other creative pursuit? Engage in activities that bring you pleasure and joy; research shows that reduces stress by almost half and lowers your heart rate, too.

Practice Meditation, Stress Reduction or Yoga: Relaxation techniques activate a state of restfulness that counterbalances your body's fight-or-flight hormones. Even if this also means a 10-minute break in a long day: listen to music, read, go for a walk in nature, do a hobby, take a bath or spend time with a friend. Also consider taking a mindfulness-based stress reduction course to learn effective, lasting tools or try a daily deep breathing or imagery practice.

Sleep Enough: If you get less than seven to eight hours of sleep, your body won't tolerate stress as well as it could. If stress keeps you up at night, address the cause and add extra meditation into your day to make up for the lost z's. Try to get seven to nine hours of sleep each night. Make a regular bedtime schedule. Keep your room dark and cool. Try to avoid computers, TV, cell phones and tablets before bed.

Bond with Connections You Enjoy: Go out for a coffee with a friend, chat with a neighbor, call a family member, visit with a clergy member, or even hang out with your pet. Clinical studies show that spending even a short time with a companion animal can cut anxiety levels almost in half.

Take a Vacation: Getting away from it all can reset your stress tolerance by increasing your mental and emotional outlook, which makes you a happier, more productive person upon return. Leave your cellphone and laptop at home!

See a Counselor, Coach or Therapist: If negative thoughts overwhelm your ability to make positive changes, it's time to seek professional help. Make an appointment today—your health and life are worth it.

# Chapter 8: Medication Management

## 8.1 Understanding Your Medications

There are many different medicines that are prescribed within the treatment of heart disease. You may have to take several different medicines every day. Though this can sometimes be difficult to deal with, try to understand and remember your doctor is aiming to keep you as well as possible and will try to find the best medicines for you with the fewest side effects.

If taking medications as directed:

- always take your medicines as prescribed by your doctor

- report any side effects but don't stop taking any medicines suddenly or without your doctor's advice

- discuss all over-the-counter remedies with your pharmacist to make sure they won't interact with any prescribed medicines you're taking. You should always tell the pharmacist and doctor/ health professional about any additional medications you're taking

- never take or "borrow" any medications prescribed for someone else

- remember drugs are often given in various combinations and are tailored to individuals. Every person may have different combinations and doses of these medications, and these may require increase or decrease in time

- any side effects or change in symptoms after you start taking a medication should be discussed with the person who prescribed them or your GP or pharmacist

- Some people sometimes forget to take their medicines. If you need help remembering to take them, talk to your doctor, pharmacist or nurse

## 8.2 Adherence and Side Effects

Managing heart disease is a multifaceted process that involves various interventions, including medications and lifestyle adjustments. One of the key determinants of success in this endeavor is patient adherence. Adherence refers to a patient's commitment to consistently following their prescribed treatment plan, which includes taking medications, adhering to dietary and exercise recommendations, and attending medical appointments. Effective heart disease management often requires long-term strategies to control risk factors and prevent complications, making adherence a vital component of the process.

Several factors influence a patient's adherence to their heart disease management plan. Understanding the importance of the treatment plan and its benefits is crucial. Simplicity and clear instructions can make adherence easier, as can having a strong social support network, including healthcare providers, family, and friends. Additionally, affordable access to prescribed medications and necessary healthcare services plays a significant role in adherence.

When these factors are optimized, patients are more likely to adhere to their treatment plans.

Medications commonly prescribed for heart disease management may have side effects, which can range from mild to severe. These side effects may include gastrointestinal issues, dizziness, fatigue, muscle pain, or changes in blood pressure. For some patients, experiencing side effects can present challenges in maintaining their treatment plan. However, not all patients will experience these effects. Open and honest communication between patients and healthcare providers is essential in addressing side effects promptly. In some cases, adjusting the medication dosage or changing to a different medication with fewer side effects may be necessary. Lifestyle modifications and regular monitoring can also help manage side effects effectively.

A comprehensive approach to improving adherence and minimizing side effects in heart disease management is essential. Patient education, providing detailed information about the disease, treatment plan, and potential side effects, helps patients understand the importance of adherence. Simplifying medication schedules and dietary guidelines can make adherence more manageable. Regular follow-up appointments with healthcare providers allow for monitoring and adjustments as needed. Encouraging patients to seek emotional support from healthcare providers, support groups, or mental health professionals can help alleviate the stress associated with managing heart disease. By addressing adherence and side effects with a patient-centered approach, healthcare teams can collaboratively work with individuals to achieve the best possible results in heart disease management.

# Chapter 9: Cardiac Rehabilitation

## 9.1 The Role of Cardiac Rehab

If you're living with heart disease, exercise may be the last thing on your mind but cardiac rehabilitation can help people with heart failure feel better and live longer. Heart failure can bring on many symptoms: shortness of breath, fatigue, swelling that makes getting through the day hard to handle. After a diagnosis, it's important to adjust your exercise, diet, and other lifestyle habits to promote heart health. That can be tough to do on your own. To help you get on track, your doctor may recommend a program known as cardiac rehabilitation, or cardiac rehab for short.

Cardiac rehab is a personalized program for people who have heart failure that's run by a team of healthcare professionals. Exercise training is the first, and most important, component of rehab. Of course, more physical activity may be the last thing on your mind. Or like others with heart failure, you may even be afraid of exerting yourself.

But a medically supervised exercise program is just what people with heart failure need, and that's not all you'll get out of cardiac rehab. These programs also teach you about nutrition, healthier choices, and how to manage your medications.

The following are the roles of a cardiac rehab:

- To improve your ability to exercise, as well as your stamina and strength

- To boost your quality of life by increasing your ability and energy to go about your day

- To lower your risk of hospitalization and death from heart failure

- To enhance  your overall psychological and social well-being by reducing stress and improving your mood

## 9.2 Participating in Your Recovery

Recovery from heart disease is a journey that demands active participation. It's not a passive process but rather a proactive commitment to one's own health. This active role empowers individuals to make informed decisions, ensures personalized care, and fosters a commitment to long-term heart health. Taking charge of your recovery is pivotal in achieving the best outcomes and a sense of control over your heart health.

Active participation empowers individuals to be informed decision-makers in their recovery journey. Understanding your heart condition and its complexities is the first step. Effective communication with your healthcare team is essential, enabling you to voice concerns and make well-informed choices about your treatment plan. Adherence to medications and treatment regimens is crucial for success, as is adopting a heart-healthy lifestyle. Equally important is understanding your medications and managing them effectively to minimize side effects.

There are practical steps individuals can take to actively participate in their heart disease recovery. Learning about your specific condition, communicating openly with your healthcare team, and following the prescribed treatment plan are foundational. Implementing heart-healthy lifestyle changes, such as diet, exercise, and stress management, is key to supporting recovery. Regular monitoring through follow-up appointments and tests ensures your progress is on track. Additionally, self-advocacy and seeking support from your social network contribute to a well-rounded approach to recovery.

Setting clear and achievable goals is a motivating factor in heart disease recovery. Collaborate with your healthcare team to define objectives such as managing cholesterol levels, reaching a healthy weight, or increasing physical activity. Tracking your progress toward these goals can instill a sense of accomplishment and motivation, reinforcing the importance of active participation in your heart health journey. With knowledge, commitment, and the support of your healthcare team and loved ones, you can actively steer your recovery toward a healthier and fulfilling life.

# Chapter 10: Survivorship and Lifestyle Beyond Heart Disease

## 10.1 Embracing a Heart-healthy Lifestyle

A healthy heart is central to overall good health. Embracing a healthy lifestyle at any age can prevent heart disease and lower your risk for a heart attack or stroke. You are never too old or too young to begin taking care of your heart. True, the younger you begin making healthy choices, the longer you can reap the benefits. But swapping good habits for bad to promote good health can make a difference, even if you've already suffered a heart attack.

Choosing healthier foods and exercising are two of the best ways to contribute to good heart health. There are additional things you can do to lower your risk for heart disease. Things that put you at higher risk for heart disease include:

- Smoking
- High blood pressure
- Obesity/being overweight
- High cholesterol levels
- Inactivity (no exercise)
- Family history of heart disease (especially a parent or sibling)

The good news is that it is possible to decrease your risk by making changes in the way you live your life. Even if you have a family history of heart disease, the power of prevention is on your side.

## 10.2 Monitoring and Preventing Recurrence

Recovery from heart disease is a significant achievement, but it doesn't mark the end of your heart health journey. To ensure your well-being and reduce the risk of recurrence, ongoing monitoring is vital. Regular check-ups, medical tests, and self-assessment are key components of this phase. It's through monitoring that you and your healthcare team can stay informed about your heart's condition and make necessary adjustments to your treatment plan. The process of monitoring is a proactive step in safeguarding your heart health.

Monitoring involves several critical aspects. Regular follow-up appointments with your healthcare team are non-negotiable. These appointments are opportunities for your cardiologist to assess your heart's condition, make any required changes to your treatment plan, and catch any issues in their early stages. Cardiac tests, such as echocardiograms and stress tests, help in evaluating your heart's function and the effectiveness of your treatment. Self-assessment is equally important; you should be attentive to your body and any unusual symptoms. Promptly reporting changes or symptoms to your healthcare provider is crucial.

Preventing the recurrence of heart disease involves a combination of lifestyle adjustments and continued adherence to your treatment plan. Medication adherence is paramount; it's essential to continue taking prescribed medications even when you're feeling well, as they play a pivotal role in managing risk factors and preventing complications. Maintaining a heart-healthy lifestyle, which includes following dietary guidelines, engaging in regular physical activity, and practicing effective stress management, is essential for long-term heart health. Smoking cessation is a top priority for those who smoke, as it significantly reduces the risk of recurrence. Weight management and stress reduction are also integral components of preventive care.

Your healthcare team is an unwavering pillar of support in preventing recurrence. They provide guidance, monitor your heart health, and offer their expertise to keep you on the path to wellness. Maintaining open communication with your healthcare team is essential. They rely on your input about any concerns, symptoms, or questions you may have. By working collaboratively with your healthcare providers and following a proactive monitoring and preventive plan, you can significantly reduce the risk of heart disease recurrence and enjoy a heart-healthy life. Your continued commitment to this journey is a testament to your dedication to your well-being.

Away from this book, it would be really appreciated if you could create time to provide a review if you thought it was worthwhile, as it would motivate me. Thanks.

www.ingramcontent.com/pod-product-compliance
Lightning Source LLC
Chambersburg PA
CBHW050843260726
48660CB00006B/2417